The Atlas of Me

The Atlas of Me

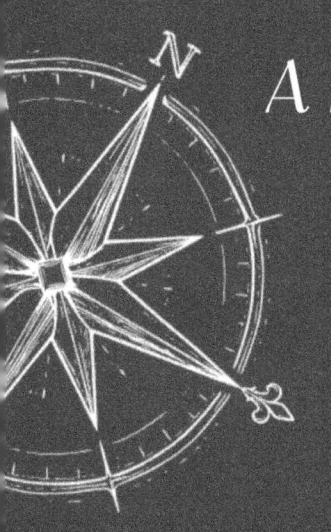

A System for Mapping Your World of Care

Developed by Tony Stewart

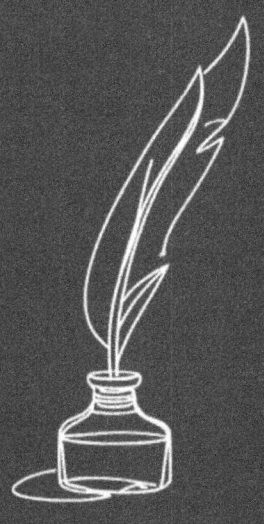

Copyright © 2025 Anthony Stewart

All rights reserved.

ISBN 978-0-646-73416-3

First published in 2026

Dedicated to my foundations

Mum

Deb Baker

Dad

Mark Henderson (1954 - 2014)

Paul & Leigh

My Flock

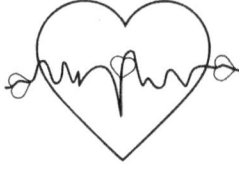

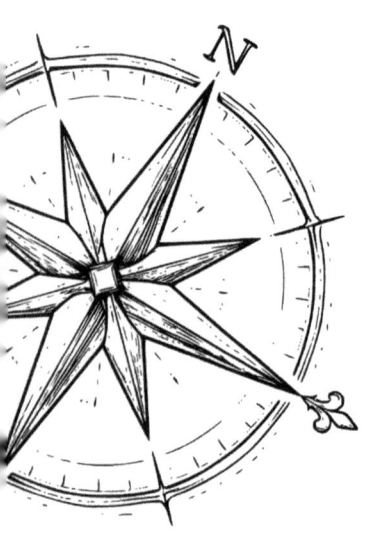

I am _____

I was born on _____

This is the Atlas of Me.

"No (Hu)man is an island,
Entire of itself;
Every (Hu)man is a piece of the continent,
A part of the main."

— John Donne

A Shifting Perspective

i. *Some Context…*
v. *Some Clarity…*
x. *Not Guidance…*
xi. *When You're Ready…*

A Guiding Perspective

1. Your Home
9. Your Yard
17. Your Neighbourhood
25. Your City
31. Your Region
37. Your Country
45. Your World

51. Travel Notes

A Classical Perspective

νθ. *Chaos*
ξα. *Enduring Wisdom*
ξγ. *Kosmos*
ξδ. *Atlas*
ξε. *Oikos*

Some Context…

Breakdowns rarely happen all at once

— they start quietly.

A task ignored. Appointments skipped, missed or cancelled. Compromises made. Small responsibilities slip because they don't feel drastically urgent.

Generally, these things hold little consequence. Over time, however, they slowly build up. Order erodes as standards fall, and our lives become chaotic.

Professional food environments understand that when our attention fragments and priorities lose focus, problems accumulate. Hygiene declines, risks increase, and the recovery effort grows.

> *A clean grill is essential, but if oil drips onto it from above and the overflow tray is full, cleaning the grill surface alone is not enough — all contributing factors need to be dealt with. The cause of the dripping, the regular cleaning of the tray, and other concerns along the chain of events requiring attention must be identified and addressed appropriately.*

To manage this, a systematic and science-based procedure is utilised.

It prompts us to think beyond the obvious surface issues, to the hidden causes and along the chain of connections beneath.

These systems are known as HACCP plans.

This acronym stands for *Hazard Analysis and Critical Control Points*, and the system was first developed for the NASA space programme.

The process uses 7 core principles:

1. *identify hazards;*
2. *determine critical points;*
3. *establish limits;*
4. *monitor procedures;*
5. *establish corrective actions;*
6. *verify processes;*
7. *maintain a progressive record.*

These plans are essential to maintaining a cohesive and systematic view. They work by generating proactive prevention from increased awareness, and are made to align with any individual approach. As a supplementary system, they also require a prior foundation of established good practices to complement.

The result is more effective and seamless daily management with less incident. A proactive awareness reduces the accumulation of problems and enhances continuity in duty of care.

When it comes to managing ourselves, we will adopt a variety of individual systems to assist us — some deliberate, many organic. What we often lack is a cohesive view across those systems.

> *Budgeting tools help with finances, diaries and planners organise our time. Journals allow visualisation of our goals, but not all important domains in our daily lives receive the same perspective.*

Fragmentation in perspective also affects our own care through daily life, and into our future.

We treat physical health here, mental health there, try to schedule exercise in between. Relationships, responsibilities, future planning, etc. — each is treated as a separate domain.

Our life moves constantly between isolated systems: stopping and starting, always reacting instead of maintaining. Regularities in life are taken for granted, thought of as merely routines and hidden by everyday familiarity.

> Gradually, our motivation drops. Care declines.
>
> The bare minimum becomes standard.
>
> Our sense of a continuous life
>
> *quietly fades away.*

Just as within professional environments, maintaining a systematic and comprehensive view of our daily life is needed. It helps to sustain our quality of life, and strengthens the connection to our living needs. We don't run our lives like businesses though — nor should we — and following such a rigid structure for ourselves would be unnecessary and excessive.

> *The perspective found by manually building these plans is where we can truly benefit from applying this to our own approach in living, and our World of Care.*

What do I mean by "World of Care"?

I define a "World of Care" as:

> *"The sphere or domain of one's life that includes providing for the needs of ourselves and others, so they are well looked after and protected in the right way."*

It encompasses all the people, responsibilities, and activities we invest our time, love, and energy into to maintain life.

Care doesn't just involve our individual needs, it extends to others that are within our World as well. When someone you care about has needs that can be supported by you, and vice versa — even if only occasionally — they're inside your World of Care.

Mundane elements like our exercise, the food we eat, or even housework are rarely considered to be a part of care. However, anything in the sphere of our lives that provides for our needs, or others connected to us, so that we are looked after, is within our World of Care.

I designed The Atlas of Me to provide a systematic approach to mapping your complete World of Care, improve self-awareness and reduce patterns of fragmentation and decline.

> *It will identify and highlight hidden connections, bring to you a higher perspective and hold a continuous record across change and boundaries.*

Map your World of Care in here and harmonise your life.

Some Clarity…

What Is "The Atlas of Me"?

A simple framework based on practical management plans used in food production. It's a re-modelling of deliberately selected procedures taken from structured business monitoring systems to a more relaxed and flexible personal care navigation system.

The objective here is not to identify hazards, roster procedures, or to plan goals. The purpose is to illuminate connections, unify daily life, and bridge gaps in care and support. This is designed to maintain continuity through life by providing a self-authored, centralised record and a systematic view of your world to supplement your own unique approach to living.

More than a decade of using similar plans has shown me the immediate and long-term benefits a cohesive structure can produce. *The Atlas of Me* can bring those benefits to your own world as you live and grow. It doesn't replace how you manage your life; it will support it by adding structure to complement your own approach.

I created *The Atlas of Me* to promote harmony and combat chaos in your World of Care. Utilising conceptual metaphor and deliberate typographic disruption to engage your mind, it provides a guided perspective and an open framework. The Atlas closes with my own philosophical perspective, inspired by Ancient Greek wisdom, before relinquishing ownership to you.

You are the centre of a small world, lay its map down here.

See the rhythm of your life, clarify your needs, and make day-to-day management easier.

Why an Atlas?

Why not a diary, journal or planner?

Diaries record events and dates.

Planners roster tasks and schedules.

Journals support reflection and emotional processing.

Life planners focus on goals and outcomes.

Self-help guides attempt to solve problems or direct behaviour.

An atlas serves a different function.

An atlas guides without instruction.

It presents a map rather than a sequence of actions.

It allows self-navigation instead of providing directions.

It shows relationships between elements across scale and time.

It has no fixed beginning or expiry date, adapting as time progresses.

This work is an atlas because it holds a living map of your World of Care — one that will evolve as your life does, and provide you with a tool for navigation without forcing a direction.

What Is Its Purpose?

To identify all your needs, recognise your care and support network, and promote a more systematic mindset towards your World of Care.

To prioritise the relative importance of all care elements in your daily and long-term life, and extend your thinking beyond individual boundaries.

To illuminate where care is interrupted when information, responsibilities and tasks are split across fragmented systems, providers, or family roles.

The Atlas of Me provides a cohesive view of your life that individual apps, lists, calendars, or reminders do not.

How Does It Work?

It clarifies your perspective on the routines, relationships and connections that maintain your stability, health, and wellbeing through daily life.

It encourages you to consider your needs more thoroughly, engages your senses through activity, and embeds knowledge deeper than memory.

It becomes a self-authored summary of important matters and changes as your World of Care evolves.

Following the mapping process provided here encourages broader thinking, and generates greater self-awareness.

What Is The Benefit?

Reassociation with all needs and support within your World of Care.

A greater awareness of connections within life, and of your future needs.

A consistent record of care and treatment to bridge change, fragmented systems, and other transitions that interrupt care throughout life.

The Atlas of Me will provide continuity, a deeper understanding, and a wider perspective to your World of Care.

Focus on your life needs, rather than goals or desires.

The Atlas of Me is about your World of Care — care meaning *"the process of providing for the needs of somebody or something, so that they are well looked after and protected in the right way"*.

Your maps may provide a clearer view of the path to achieving your goals, or you might find new objectives to reach for through the perspective the Atlas gives you. Adding them here though will only create unnecessary detours.

Aspirations and dreams are necessary, but this is not the place to keep track of those things.

This is not a system to optimise your life.

It is not a plan to follow,
nor a checklist to complete.

It is a self-built map of your world

— no more, no less.

There are no laws in here.

No prescribed methods.

No borrowed wisdom or self-improvement advice.

This is only a frame around an empty canvas.

Map your world for yourself — written by your own hand, and in your own time.

Not Guidance…

The first thing to keep in mind is:

There are no rules

There is no correct way to use this.

There is no wrong way to use this!

There is only your way

— your pace, your style, your voice.

No exam awaits you. There's no time limit. No final score.

Add to it, change it, modify it over time.

The aim is to do this thoughtfully, not quickly.

Fill in some, or all.

Express your style!

Doodle, *improvise*, or be meticulous.

If you're unsure, do whatever feels right.

It's entirely up to you.

This is made for your hands, not a programmed structure.

Fill this empty canvas.

Build your own map on it.

When You're Ready...

Grab your favourite pen.

                        Find a comfortable seat.

                                        Relax your mind.

                                                          Slow your pace.

Consider each perspective individually.
                              Map one domain at a time.

The Atlas of Me reveals itself gradually, progressively assembling into a complete picture as your perspective moves towards the horizon.

When building each perspective map, consider the tables as paved yet unnamed streets ready for a new neighbourhood.

                         The lines define paths and boundaries only.

You build the houses, name the roads, choose which to travel down, and decide how far they reach.

                    The only direction is to think outside the lines.

Broaden your view.

                      Ask one more question.

                                        Engage your mind.

As you go, consider each thing and ask:

Do I care about this?

Can I live without it?

What do I need to maintain it?

What else affects this, for better or worse?

How would I feel if I couldn't have it?

When identifying your care support network, ask:

Does, or can, this person's support help with my needs?

Does, or can, my support help with their needs?

What do I need to know about them, or them about me?

Do I rely on them? Do they rely on me?

These are only suggestions to get you started and to prompt more lateral thinking, while anchoring your perspective in care. With the priorities in focus, this is a simple process which encourages a wider perspective.

Don't feel overwhelmed — you won't think of everything the first time.

Include the obvious now. Return later to add layers as new considerations and connections emerge.

You are the World in this Atlas.

Know thyself.

The Atlas begins in the year: 20____

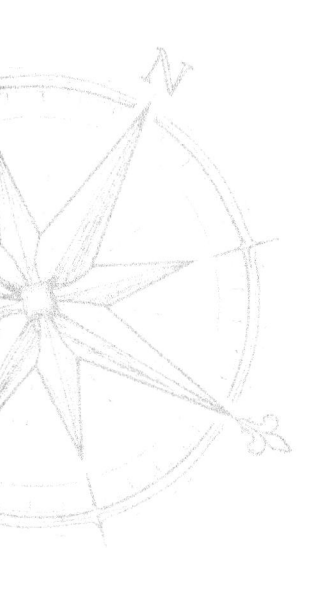

Perspective Guidance
Your Home

Begin with those who connect to your personal network of care: family, pets, exercise partners, supportive co-workers or friends — anyone relevant to your daily living needs.

If they regularly support you, or rely on your support, include them here.

Including their relationship to you, age, and life stage adds context.

Some suggestions to define life stages:

New Life: 0–2, Toddler: 2–4

Early Life: 4–8, Tween: 8–12

Teenage: 12–20, Early Adulthood: 20–30

Partnership: 25–40 or Parenthood: 25–40

Maturity: 30 – 40, Mid-Life: 40–55

Retirement: 55–70, Late Life: 70+

Use any terms you like here —

Sprog, Young & Dumb, Silverback

— the choice is yours, have fun with it.

This is not a clinical record, it's a summary and overview.

This is the foundation your Atlas builds on.

Your World of Care is centred here.

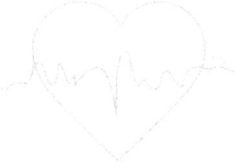

Note any significant health and wellbeing priorities.

These may include dietary, exercise or mobility needs, medical, physical or mental health considerations, sensory or behavioural patterns

— *anything influencing daily stability and wellbeing.*

Important contacts sit alongside this view

to unify your needs and support channels.

Add the professionals, services, organisations,

and personal or community contacts you rely on.

Together, these pages create a picture of your home — your family and friends within, the ground beneath it, and the sheltering walls.

This is where your worldview radiates from, growing with each step through the maps of your Atlas.

Home Map
Personal Care Ecosystem

Immediate Family

Name　　　　　　　　*Relation*　　　　　*Birth Year*　　　　*Life Stage*

_____

_____

_____

_____

_____

_____

_____

_____

_____

_____

_____

_____

_____

_____

_____

_____

_____

_____

_____

Home Map
Extended Care Ecosystem

Extended Support Family

Name	Relation	Birth Year	Life Stage

Home Map
Ecosystem Care Priorities

Medical & Health Priority Details

Name	Health	Medical	Other Care

Home Map
Ecosystem Support Contacts

Support Contacts

Contact Name   *Organisation*   *Details*

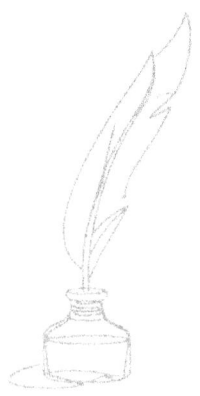

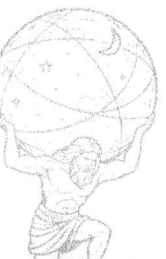

Perspective Guidance
Your Yard

Your Yard represents those things closest to Home that maintain life, help you manage day-to-day, and operate in the world beyond your gates.

Keep your mind open as you step beyond the Home Perspective.

Mapping your Yard requires reflection and deliberate thinking.

Take your time.

Return later if you wish.

There is no need to do everything now.

Through this perspective, identify daily care needs.

They may be simple or detailed, regular or occasional.

Include the essentials such as medications, morning routines, personal hygiene, or meals, as well as any activities that support focus and wellbeing — caring for children or pets, exercise, meditation, or anything else that stabilises your day.

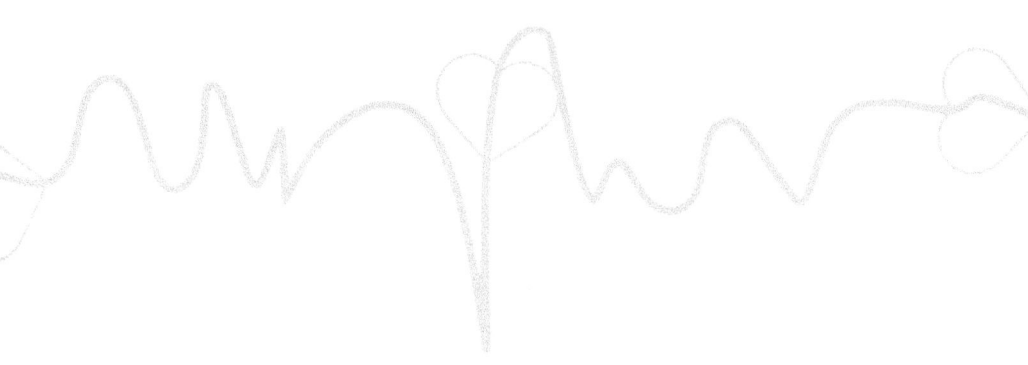

Determine your priorities in a way that makes sense to you.

One useful approach is to distinguish between what you need, want, or simply like to have on a daily basis.

This clarifies what requires special attention, what is essential, and where you can allow flexibility.

The following pages

— *Morning, Day, and Night* —

lay out the rhythm of your daily life.

This is the second foundational step and illuminates what influences stability in daily life.

As you reach your gates, the path ahead begins to move into the areas of your world visited less often.

Yard Map
Personal Daily Priorities

I Need To Have

I Want To Have

I Like To Have

Yard Map
Family Daily Priorities

We Need To Have

_____   _____
_____   _____
_____   _____
_____   _____
_____   _____
_____   _____
_____   _____
_____   _____

We Want To Have

_____   _____
_____   _____
_____   _____
_____   _____
_____   _____

We Like To Have

_____   _____
_____   _____
_____   _____
_____   _____
_____   _____

Yard Map
Personal Daily Routine

Morning

Day

Night

Yard Map
Family Daily Routine

Morning

Day

Night

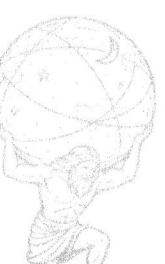

Perspective Guidance
Your Neighbourhood

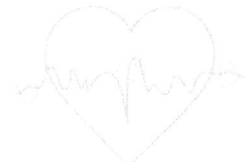

Now that the foundational areas of your World are mapped, what follows becomes easier.

This chapter extends
                the same thinking
                              into a wider scope.

Your neighbourhood includes the regular weekly care routines, activities and responsibilities that don't occur daily

but remain habitual or necessary.

Use these pages as before: note what matters, rank priorities, and distribute them across the week to suit your schedule.

There is nothing new to learn from here — you have all of the understanding of the method you now need.

Repeat the process at your own pace.

Keep thinking broadly.

Let the structure support you, not rush you.

This step adds the secondary roads to less regularly visited locations branching from your most often travelled highways and stops.

The hard part is done.

Now you are simply adding more detail to your map.

Neighbourhood Map

Personal Weekly Priorities

I Need To Have

_____   _____
_____   _____
_____   _____
_____   _____
_____   _____
_____   _____
_____   _____
_____   _____

I Want To Have

_____   _____
_____   _____
_____   _____
_____   _____

I Like To Have

_____   _____
_____   _____
_____   _____
_____   _____
_____   _____

Neighbourhood Map
Family Weekly Priorities

We Need To Have

We Want To Have

We Like To Have

Neighbourhood Map
Weekly Routine

Monday

Tuesday

Wednesday

Neighbourhood Map
Weekly Routine

Thursday

Friday

Weekends

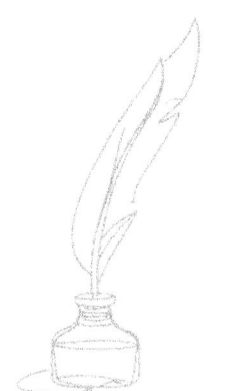

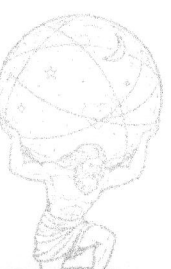

Perspective Guidance
Your City

This chapter broadens your view further.

Your City represents the monthly tasks that don't require constant attention, but benefit from being seen and planned for intentionally.

The structure is familiar now.

Continue with the same process and
                      extend your thinking over a longer distance.

Note tasks, needs, or commitments that stabilise you monthly.

Add dates, or don't, use your own discretion.

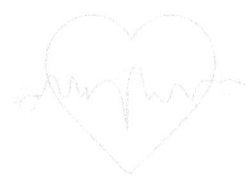

Here, your Atlas begins to reveal less obvious patterns within your immediate sphere.

Notice where conflicts occur. Consider how the longer paths of your daily life can influence the smaller steps. Does something need more support or regularity? Is anything interrupted by other routines?

From this point you can begin to see if there are more efficient routes to take between the different locations you visit.

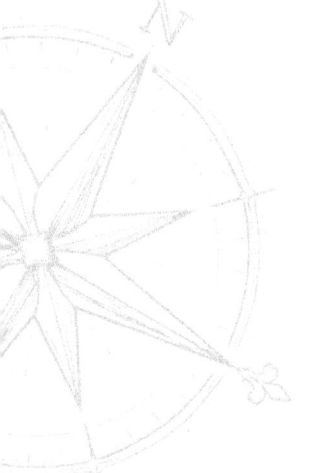

You've done the hard work now.

These downhill steps will be lighter,

with less effort.

Let the process flow naturally as your Atlas continues to assemble.

City Map

Personal Monthly Priorities

I Need To Have   *Date*

_____

_____

_____

_____

_____

_____

_____

_____

I Want To Have   *Date*

_____

_____

_____

_____

I Like To Have   *Date*

_____

_____

_____

_____

City Map
Family Monthly Priorities

We Need To Have   *Date*

_____ _____

_____ _____

_____ _____

_____ _____

_____ _____

_____ _____

_____ _____

We Want To Have   *Date*

_____ _____

_____ _____

_____ _____

_____ _____

We Like To Have   *Date*

_____ _____

_____ _____

_____ _____

_____ _____

_____ _____

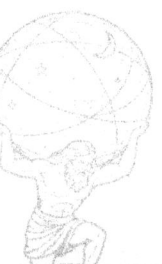

Perspective Guidance
Your Region

Your regional perspective ascends above the domains that you've mapped so far.

Previous views were from ground level.

Now the path rises,

to reveal the wider landscape.

Define the tasks, milestones, and responsibilities that occur throughout the year — the elements that stabilise your life annually.

Detail is not required;

simply note what matters.

This map completes the view of your familiar land.

As you explore this annual layer, notice again how the more immediate aspects of your life interrelate with the less regular elements.

With your home territory mapped, the next pages invite you to raise your perspective further

— *toward the destinations ahead.*

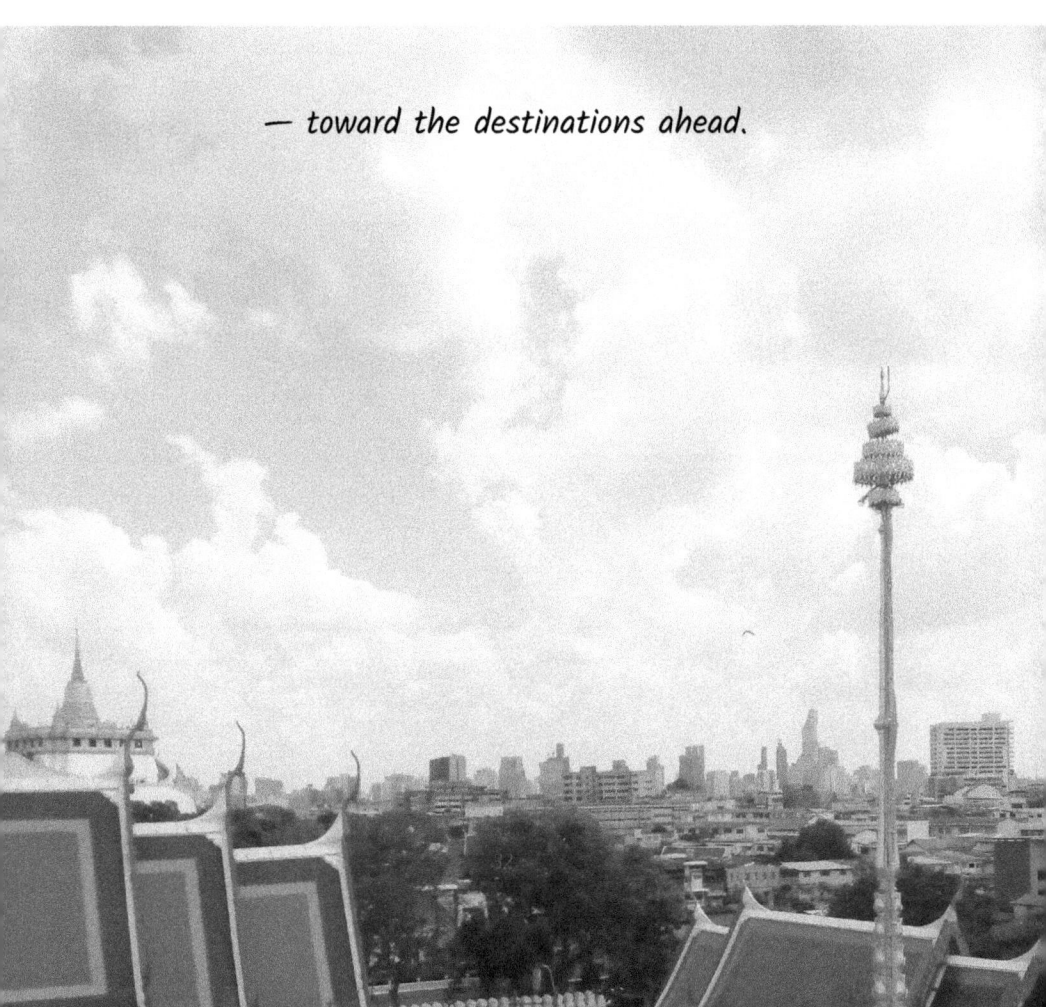

Regional Map

Personal Annual Priorities

I Need To Have   *Month*

I Want To Have   *Month*

I Like To Have   *Month*

Regional Map
Family Annual Priorities

We Need To Have _Month_

_____ _____
_____ _____
_____ _____
_____ _____
_____ _____
_____ _____
_____ _____

We Want To Have _Month_

_____ _____
_____ _____
_____ _____
_____ _____

We Like To Have _Month_

_____ _____
_____ _____
_____ _____
_____ _____

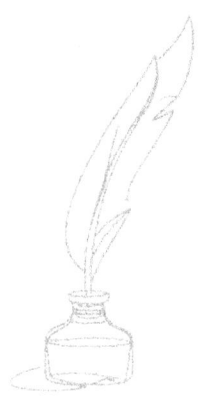

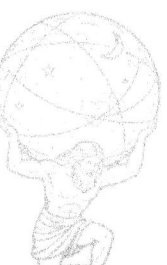

Perspective Guidance
Your Country

The Next Five Years

Look to the horizon now, and consider what approaches.

Over the coming years, certain needs, changes, or milestones may arise

— for you or those you support.

Health checks, growth and school transitions, family and developmental shifts, and other one-time occurrences shape our life — *whether planned or not.*

This step is not about aspirations or goals.

It's about acknowledging what is likely to come —

things we know are ahead, *but rarely prepare for.*

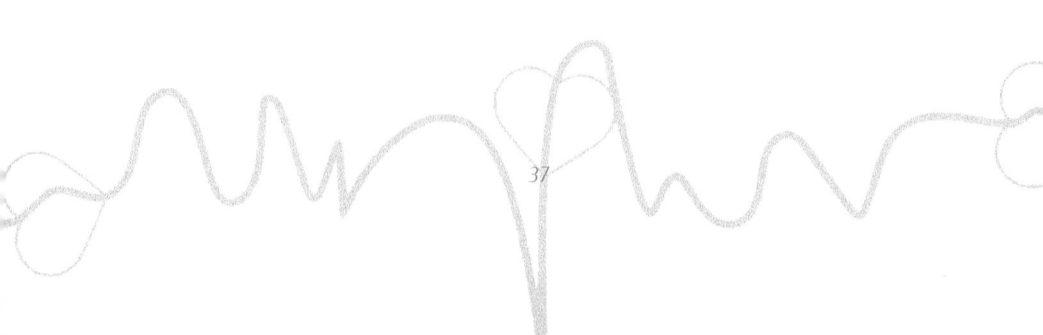

Climb to a stratospheric level now.

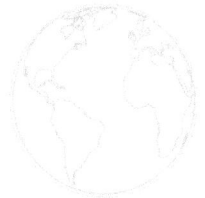

Look ahead and mark the mountains you may climb, the borders you may cross, the destinations you may reach.

Precision is not required.

The future is not fixed

— nor is this view.

And that's OK.

Your Atlas will provide you a continuous path through unfamiliar terrain, and will become a reliable map as you travel forward.

Looking 5 years ahead from: 20___

Country Map
Personal Care Preparations

Event *Next Year: 20___* *Month*

_____
_____
_____
_____
_____
_____
_____
_____
_____
_____

Event *2 Years Ahead: 20___* *Month*

_____
_____
_____
_____
_____
_____
_____
_____
_____
_____

Country Map

Personal Care Preparations

| Event | 3 Years Ahead: 20___ | Month |

_____
_____
_____
_____
_____
_____

| Event | 4 Years Ahead: 20___ | Month |

_____
_____
_____
_____
_____
_____

| Event | 5 Years Ahead: 20___ | Month |

_____
_____
_____
_____
_____
_____

Country Map
Family Care Preparations

Event *Next Year: 20___* *Month*

_____
_____
_____
_____
_____
_____
_____
_____
_____
_____

Event *2 Years Ahead: 20___* *Month*

_____
_____
_____
_____
_____
_____
_____
_____
_____
_____

Country Map
Family Care Preparations

Event *3 Years Ahead: 20___* *Month*

_____
_____
_____
_____
_____
_____

Event *4 Years Ahead: 20___* *Month*

_____
_____
_____
_____
_____
_____

Event *5 Years Ahead: 20___* *Month*

_____
_____
_____
_____
_____
_____

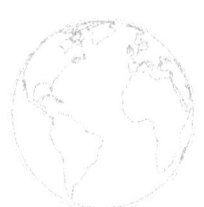

Perspective Guidance
Your World

The Long Journey

This is a quiet space to consider the future route and any distant landmarks along your road.

Two decades will give you an adequate time-frame to acknowledge any approaching certainties and possibilities that matter.

Note what is certain to occur.

Life changes or retirement.

Children leaving school or home.

Other major life transitions.

Don't predict outcomes or create plans here.

This is not a wish or bucket list.

Think of this as a rough outline
of lands not yet visited.

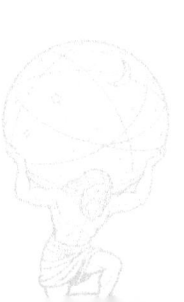

The map now extends beyond your visible horizon.

Few details are enough —

add more as they emerge

It's not about predicting,

it's about acknowledging.

The future is certain to change, as are you.

This is The Atlas of **You** now.

It maps the paths you walk,

the territories you cross,

and the world you navigate.

Looking to the Horizon from: 20 ____

World Map
Personal Care Preparations

Event   *My Horizon: 20___ to 20___*   *Year*

_____

_____

_____

_____

_____

_____

_____

_____

Event   *Beyond My Horizon: 20___ to 20___*   *Year*

_____

_____

_____

_____

_____

_____

_____

_____

_____

_____

World Map
Family Care Preparations

Event   *Our Horizon: 20___ to 20___*   *Year*

_____

_____

_____

_____

_____

_____

_____

_____

Event   *Beyond Our Horizon: 20___ to 20___*   *Year*

_____

_____

_____

_____

_____

_____

_____

_____

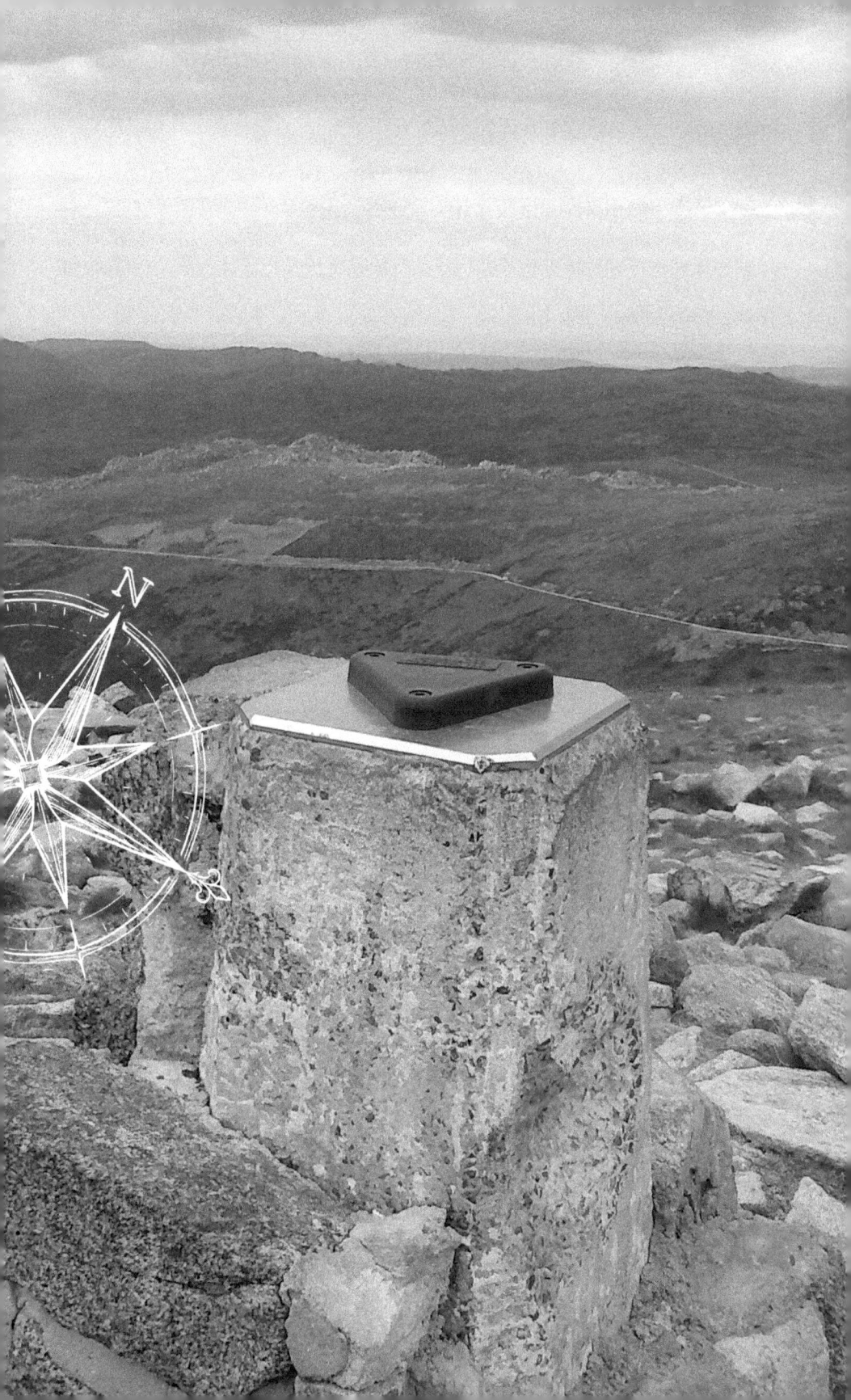

Travel Notes

Your Atlas carries an evolving view of your World of Care, mapped as one harmonious ecosystem —

From your Home Yard, to a satellite perspective of your World.

Built on your foundations, written by your hand, this world is populated with your people, and sustains your life. Its coastlines are formed by the rhythm of your tides, lands defined by your changing needs, and dawn rises to your routine.

This will never be complete — it's made to change with your life — but through this process you have mapped your Atlas to the edges of your World of Care.

What Now?

Move forward with a higher awareness and deeper understanding of what keeps the rhythm of your life steady. See more clearly where care can be improved in your world. Learn where fragmentation interrupts daily life, use this to maintain continuity, and to balance you from day to day.

Take this new mindset forward with you, and update your maps as needs change. Revisit your Atlas to spend time with yourself, quiet the noise, and strengthen the tactile connection to your world.

These final pages are your space.

Use them however you wish.

This is
The Atlas of You.

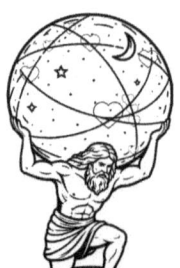

Travel Notes

Note *Date*

Travel Notes

Note *Date*

Travel Notes

Note *Date*

Travel Notes

Note *Date*

Travel Notes

Note *Date*

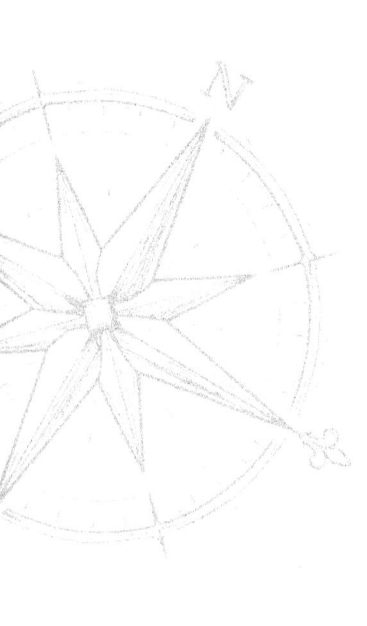

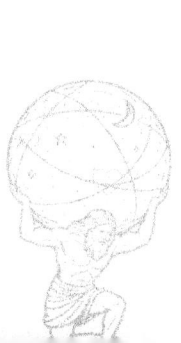

Chaos

Do you still hear your own voice?

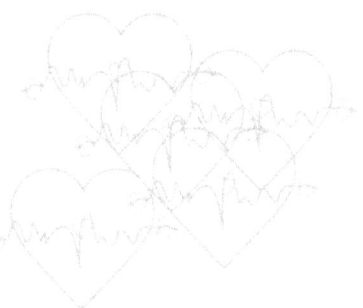

Are you choosing — or being influenced?

As modern solutions multiply, do you still feel in control?

Setting reminders to check trackers.

Getting notifications about reminders.

Scheduling alarms just to keep up.

At what point does this become more noise
           and just another thing to manage?

**And will AI distance us even further,
as it promises more time for life?**

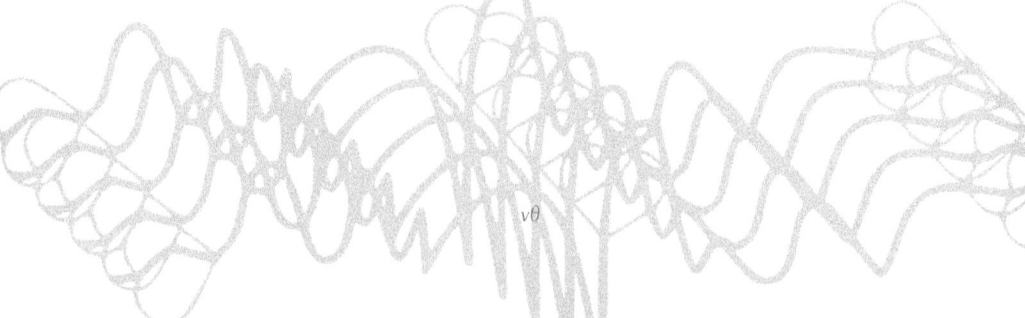

We track the minutiae of life

      while losing track of ourselves.

Tactile anchors to reality

— to our sensory world —

are becoming essential.

So too are reasons to listen to our own thoughts.

This is a physical book
to meet that need and reduce the *chaos*.

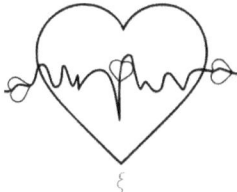

Enduring Wisdom

Engaging with your Atlas restores a tactile connection to your world and re-invigorates the senses.

>The action stimulates neural pathways producing measurable health benefits.

Writing activates the mind,

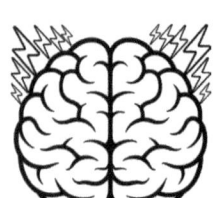

focuses attention,

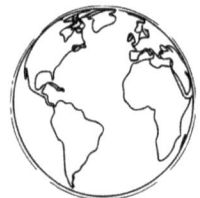

and grounds you in the present.

Socrates believed the mental friction we produce from the effort of thinking — discovering understanding for oneself — is a more effective method of learning than hearing or reading answers.

Increasingly, we see the effects modern life is having on our health, mental focus and brain development, particularly among younger generations. We often return to traditional ways only after suffering from the loss of things once taken for granted.

Small acts
— like picking up a pen and taking time to think —
can have a meaningful impact.

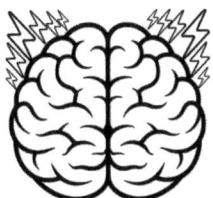

It is not about generating words,
it's about encoding knowledge through action.

Creating thoughts from scratch engages multiple regions of the brain simultaneously, embedding information more deeply.

This is known as the Generation Effect.

Feel the world you inhabit.
Keep your mind active.

Using your Atlas strengthens your connection to life, reducing the volume on the noise of algorithms and digital systems.

Quiet the noise. Hear your own voice.
Listen to yourself before another app or program.

Kosmos

In Ancient Greece, *Kosmos* defines a cohesive world as one system balancing unity, beauty, and function in complete harmony.

Kosmos is the polar opposite of *Chaos*.

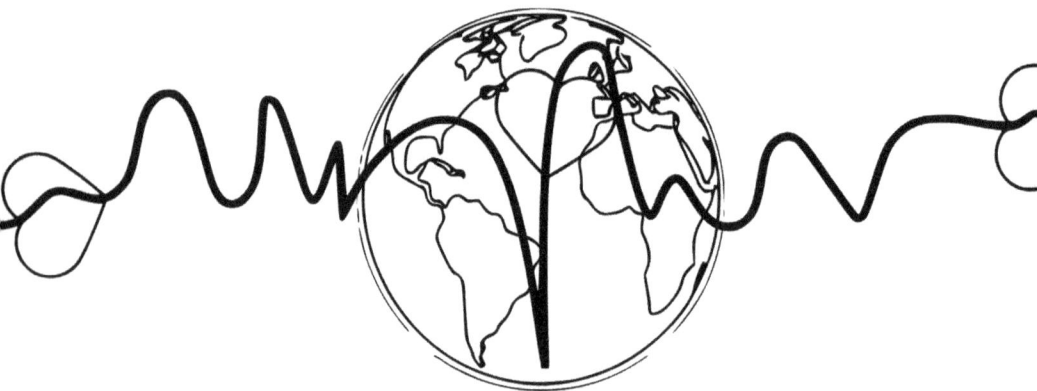

Harmony still exists through our world, but we drown under the noise of increasing chaos. In that dissonance, our lives fragment — *and we suffer.* When fragmentation interrupts continuous care, consequences ripple through our health, relationships, future wellbeing and more.

Restoring and maintaining harmony in our lives requires a cohesive view of the system.

Atlas

The Atlas of Me is designed to interrupt noise, reduce the dissonance, bridge divides and maintain harmony.

It holds a higher perspective of your world and will become a living record you can revisit, evolving as your needs change.

When life feels unmanageable —

and it seems the sky is falling

— your Atlas will support it.

This is not only a map.

Like the mythological Atlas with the Celestial Sphere on his shoulders, this Atlas will lift some of the burden from yours, and support your life at ground level through time and change.

This is not a life guide you follow — *your Atlas will follow you.*

It will help you to maintain continuity through change, and carry some of your cognitive load.

Oikos

Life requires many forms of care — some small and immediate, some steady and familiar, others emerging across years. Rarely do we see all of our needs as a cohesive system, so naturally, we struggle with consistent management through interruptions and over time.

Working through these pages, you've built a clear map of that system — your World of Care, or *Kosmos*.

Through engagement with this active process, you've generated enduring wisdom. With deeper understanding, you will rely less on memory. With more awareness of the patterns in your life, care will be more proactive and control will return to you.

In business environments these systems are used to monitor and maintain — *not replace* — established approaches to management. They include monitoring, correcting, and verifying the procedures and outcomes, while supporting and supplementing existing practices.

***The Atlas of Me* is the system map of your World of Care — the practice and approach is entirely in your hands.**

You've built your personal living Atlas now.

The Atlas of Me does not tell you who to be, or how to live.

It carries your *Kosmos* through change and across boundaries.

It helps you to navigate a continuous course through life.

Return here whenever you need —

to ground yourself, reconnect, and update your World of Care.

Include a reminder to revisit your Atlas from time to time, perhaps in your monthly or annual chapter. Use it as a tool to hear your voice and relax.

This companion will evolve with you, support your life, and remain steady through a changing world. I hope the understanding you've built here strengthens your path.

Travel forward, your Atlas will be a constant.

Let it clarify your life and navigate the road ahead.

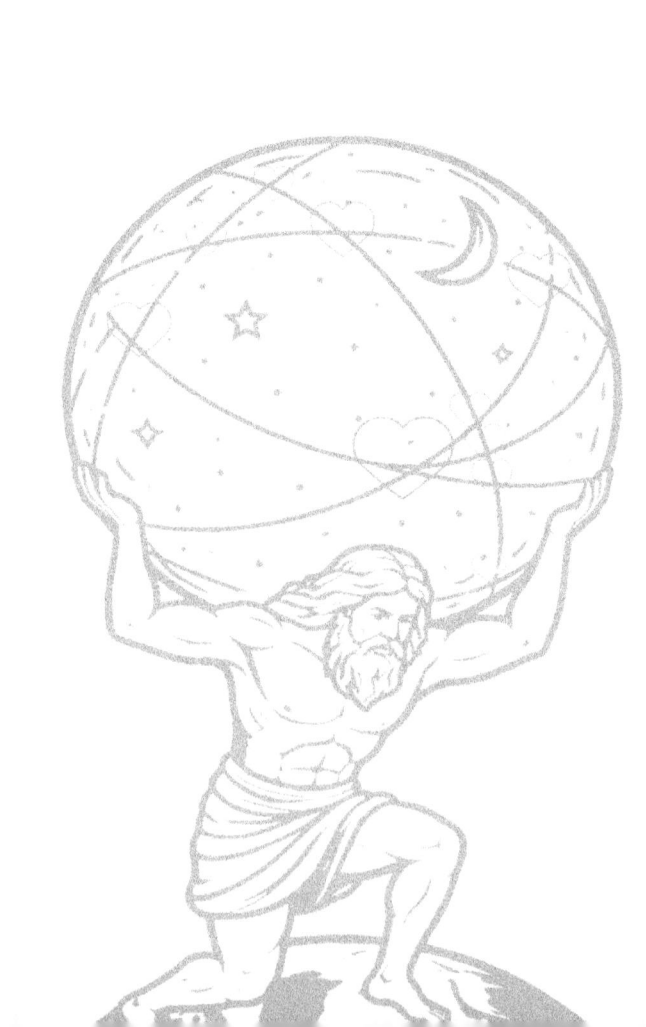

About the Designer

Tony Stewart has spent more than three decades working in hospitality and food production, with over fifteen years' experience as a certified Food Safety Supervisor. His professional life has regularly involved designing, implementing, and maintaining systems that ensure continuity across complex, high-pressure environments.

Through years of working with structured frameworks such as food safety and quality control plans, he became increasingly interested in how the same principles can be applied to everyday life — most particularly where fragmentation, cognitive overload, and loss of perspective undermine our care and wellbeing.

The Atlas of Me: A System for Mapping Your World of Care emerged from the intersection of professional practice, lived experience, and an interest in philosophy and systems thinking. It was designed as a physical tool to help restore connection, continuity, and perspective to life.

Tony lives in Australia with his small flock of parrots.

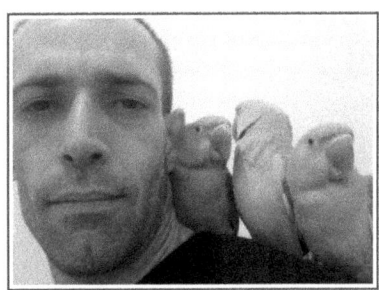

The Atlas of Me was designed by Tony Stewart,

but you are its Author.

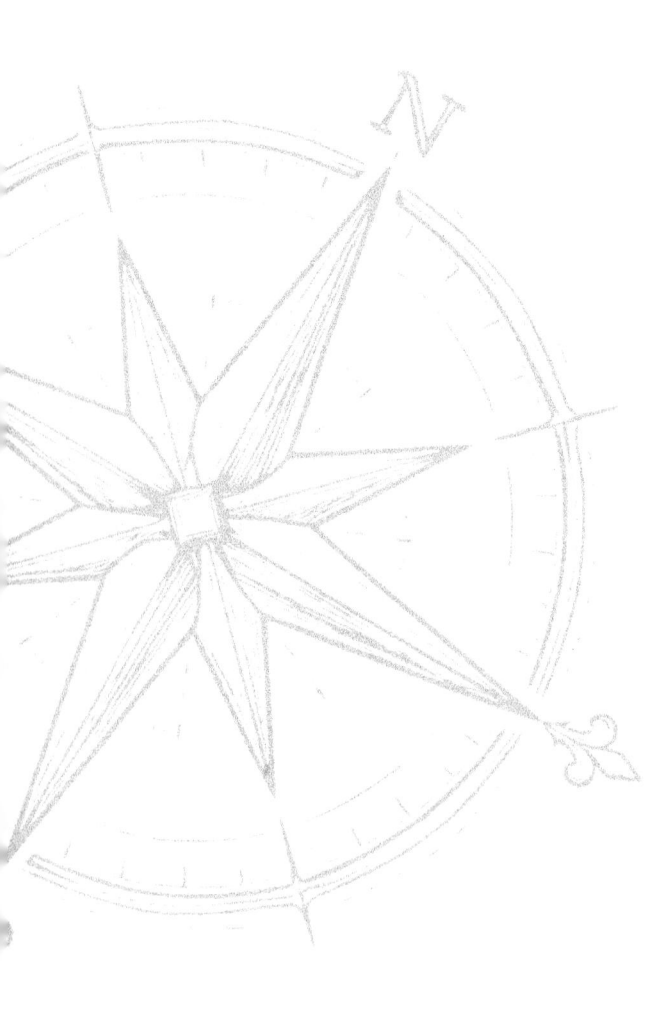